Elephant Playground Incident

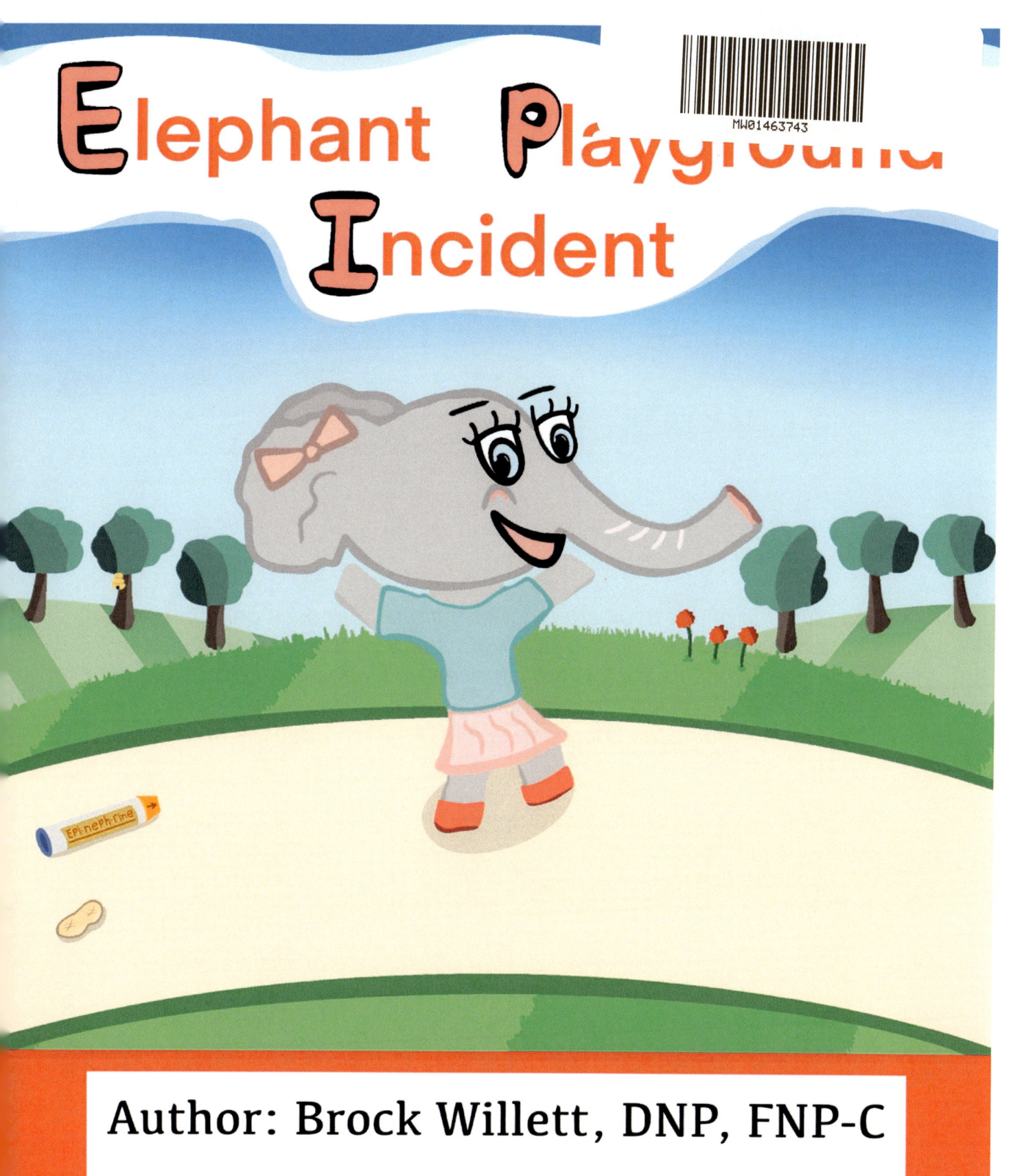

Author: Brock Willett, DNP, FNP-C

Illustrator: Vittorio Nocera

The contents of this book are for informational purposes only and are not intended to diagnose, treat, cure, or prevent any condition or disease. You understand that this book is not intended as a substitute for consultation with a licensed practitioner. Please consult with your own healthcare provider regarding the suggestions and recommendations made in this book.

The author and the illustrator advise you to take full responsibility for your safety and know your limits. Before practicing the skills described in this book, be sure that your equipment is well maintained and do not take risks beyond your level of experience, aptitude, training, and comfort level..

The use of this book implies your acceptance of this disclaimer.

Baby EL put on your shoes.

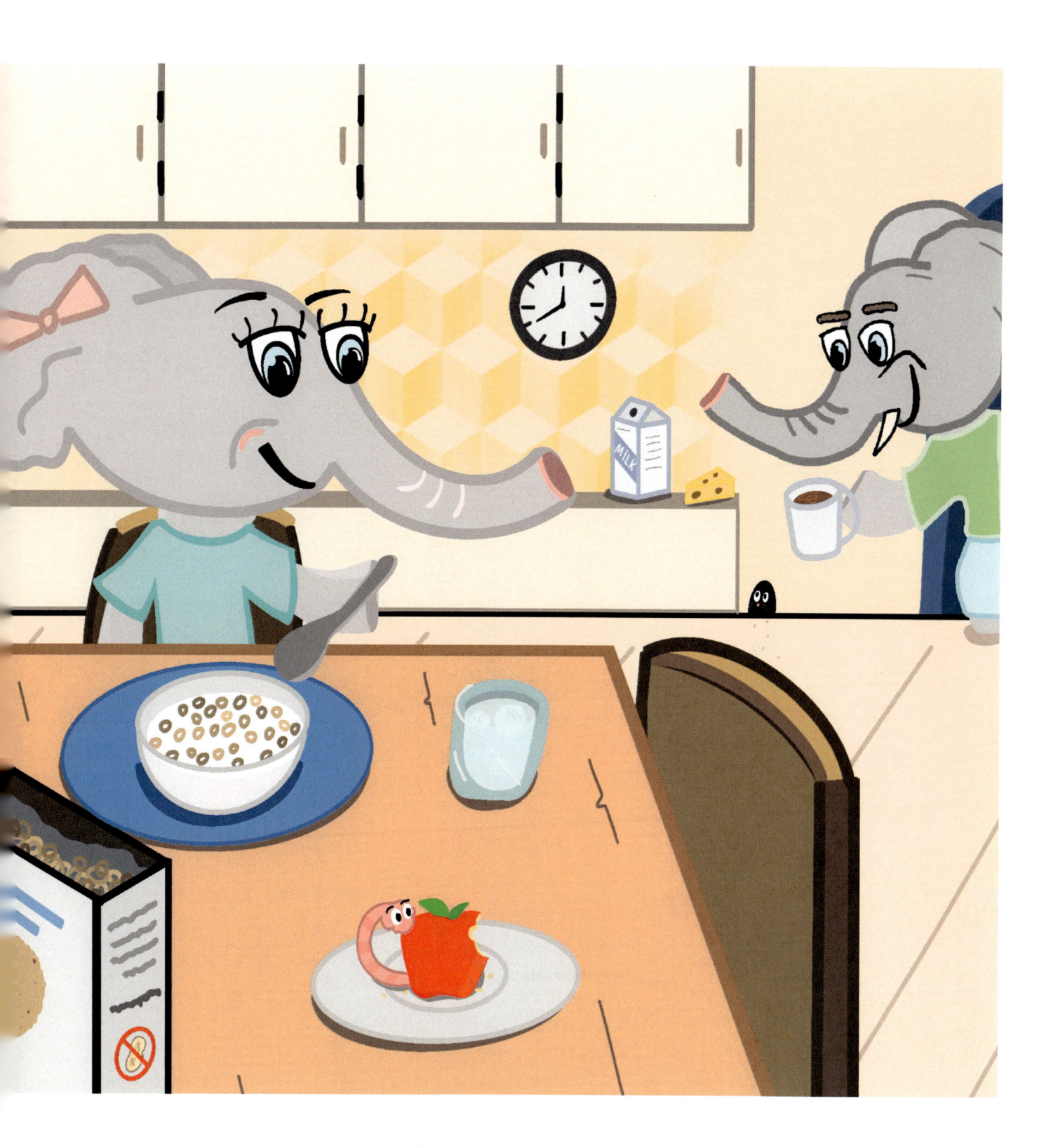

We are going to the park after I finish watching the news.

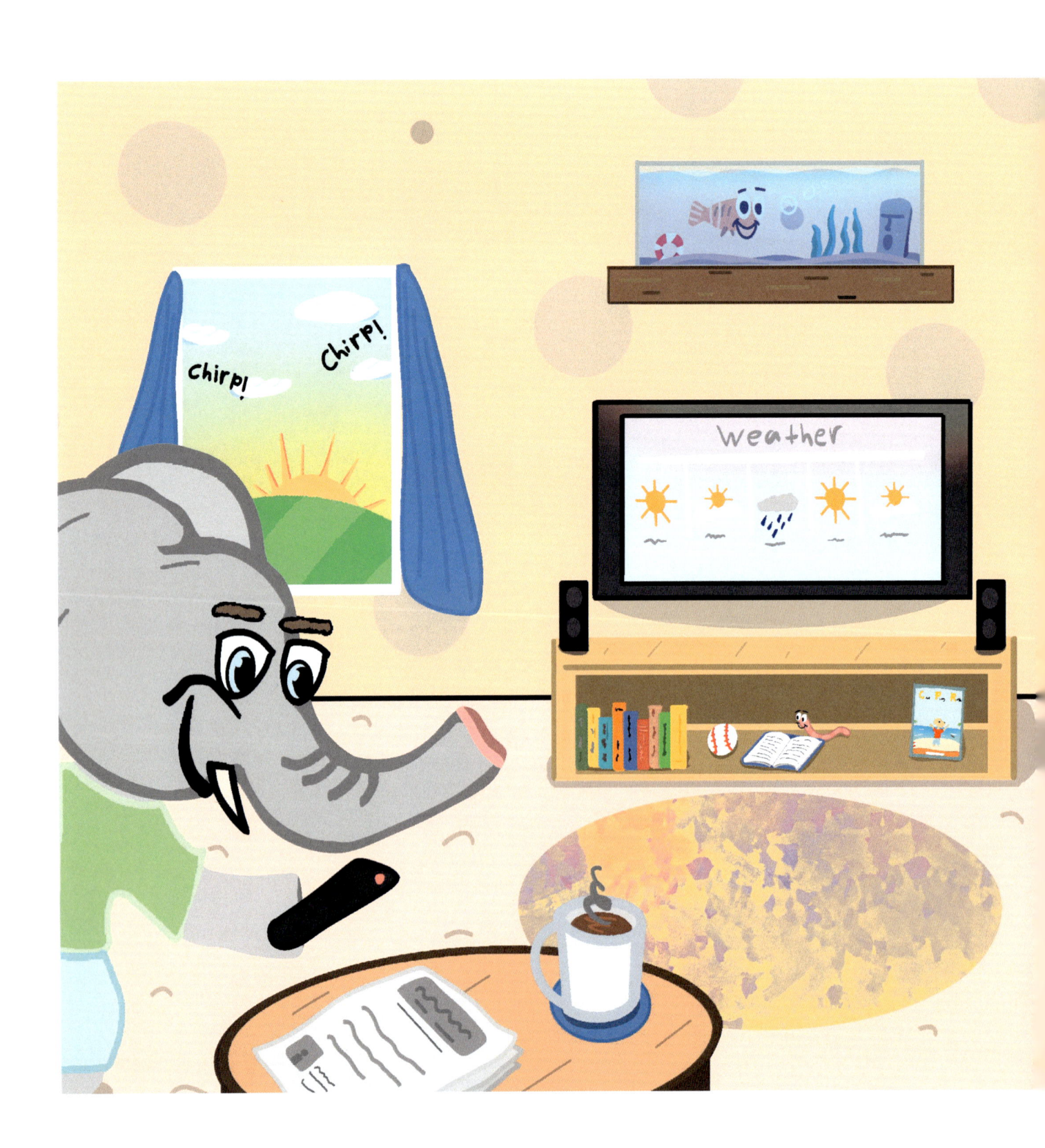

To the playground we shall go.

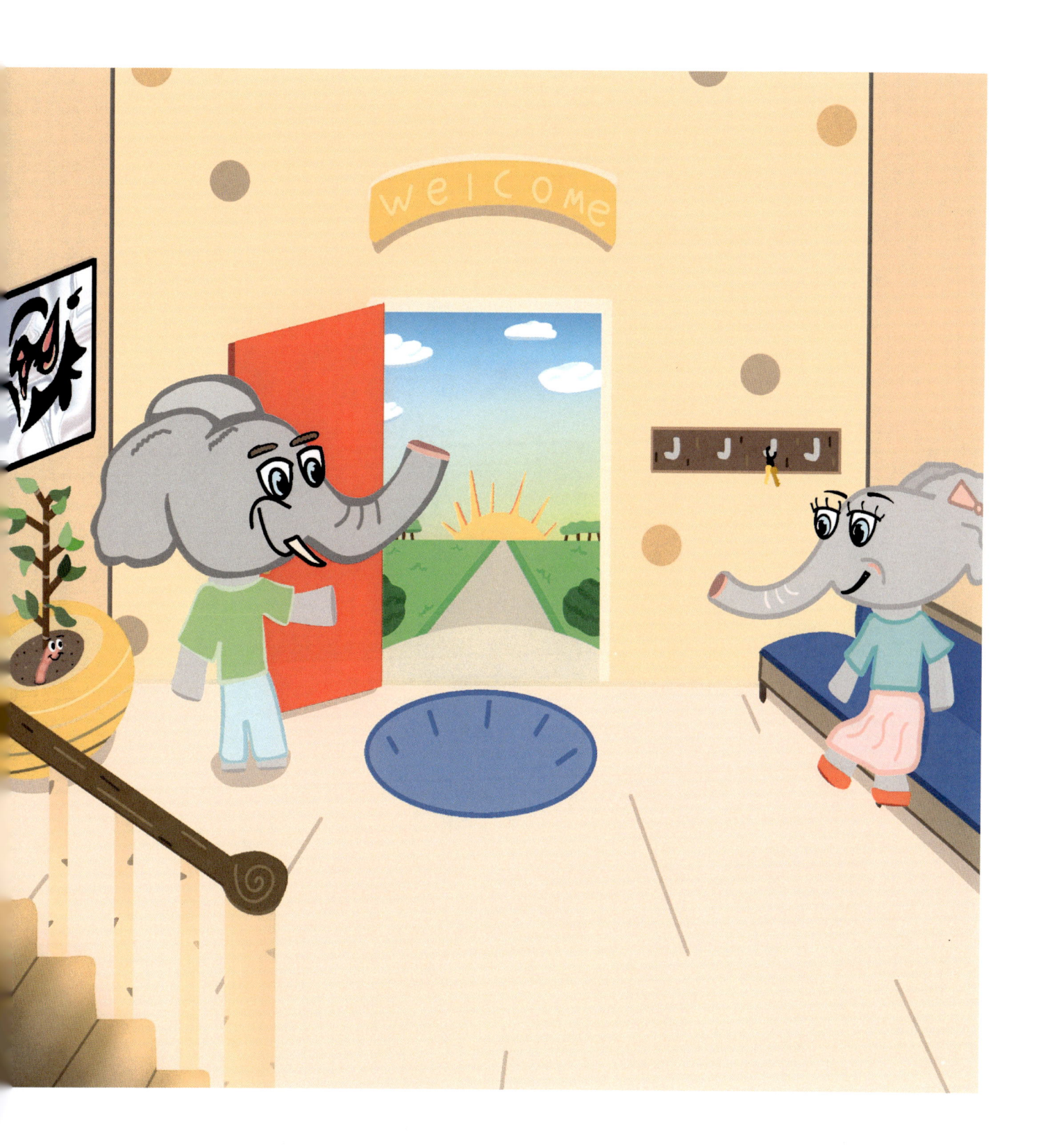

Let's wave to our neighbor, buffalo Joe.

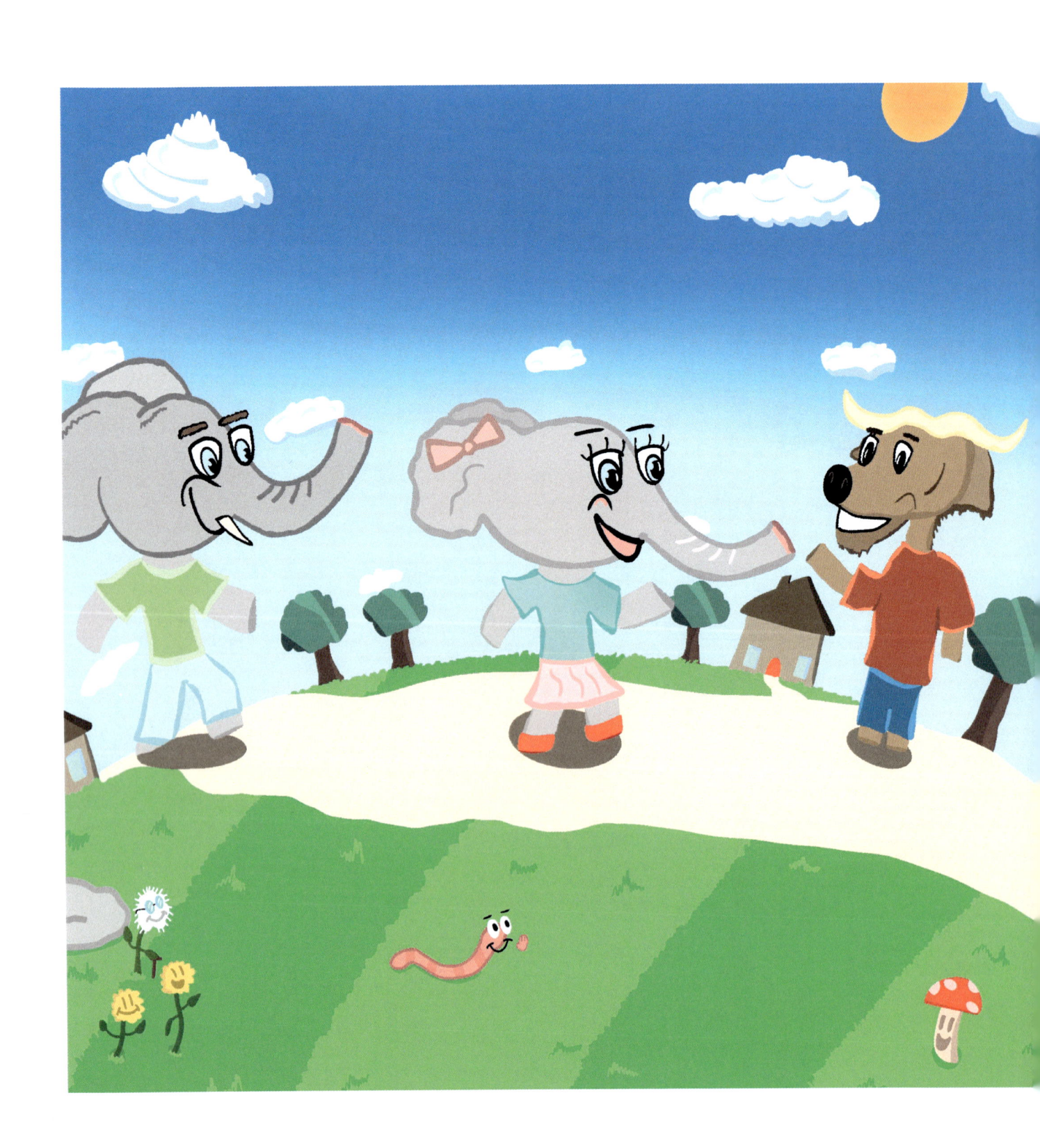

The playground has so many colors!

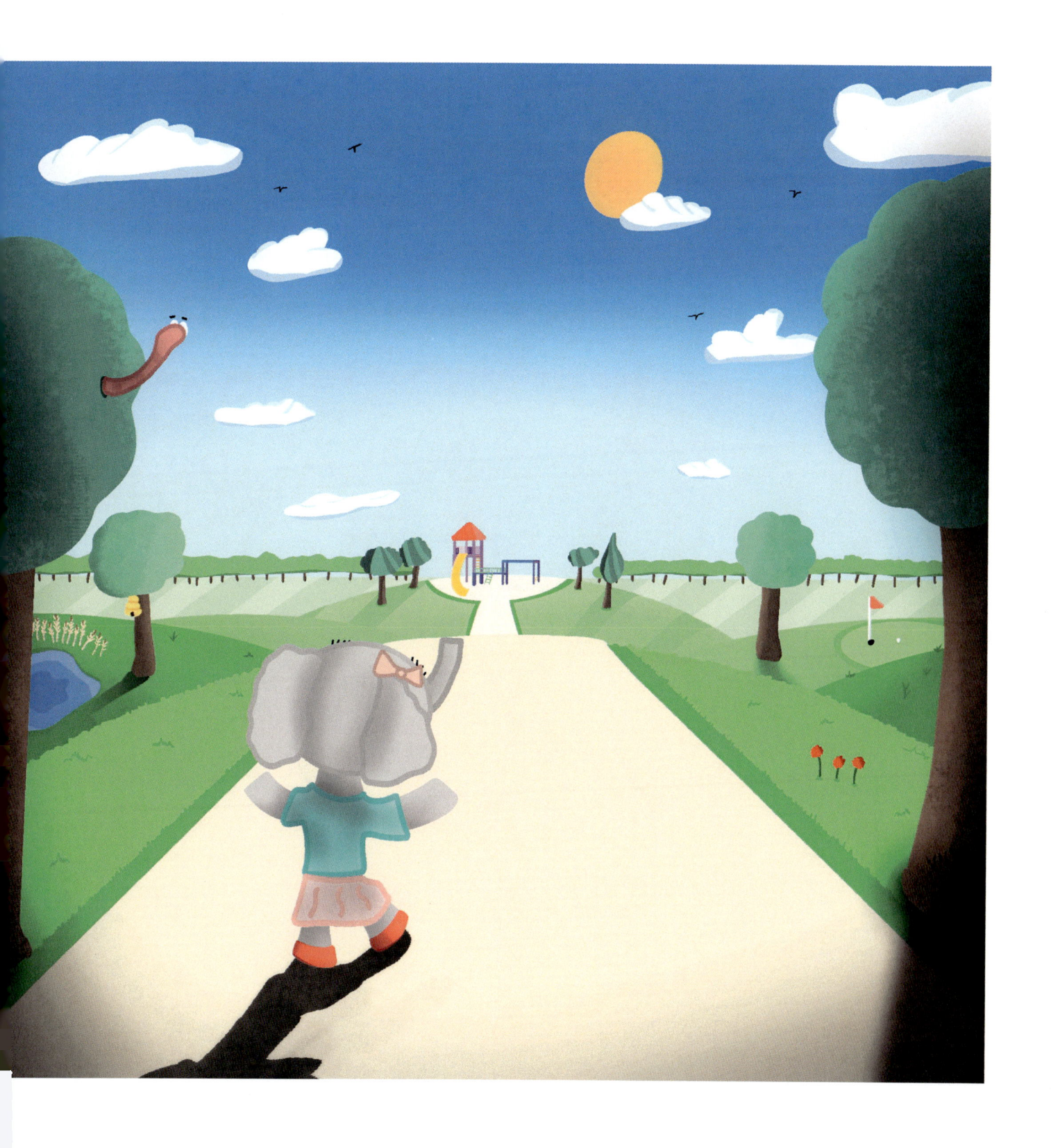

Hey, look!

There's my best friend with her brothers.

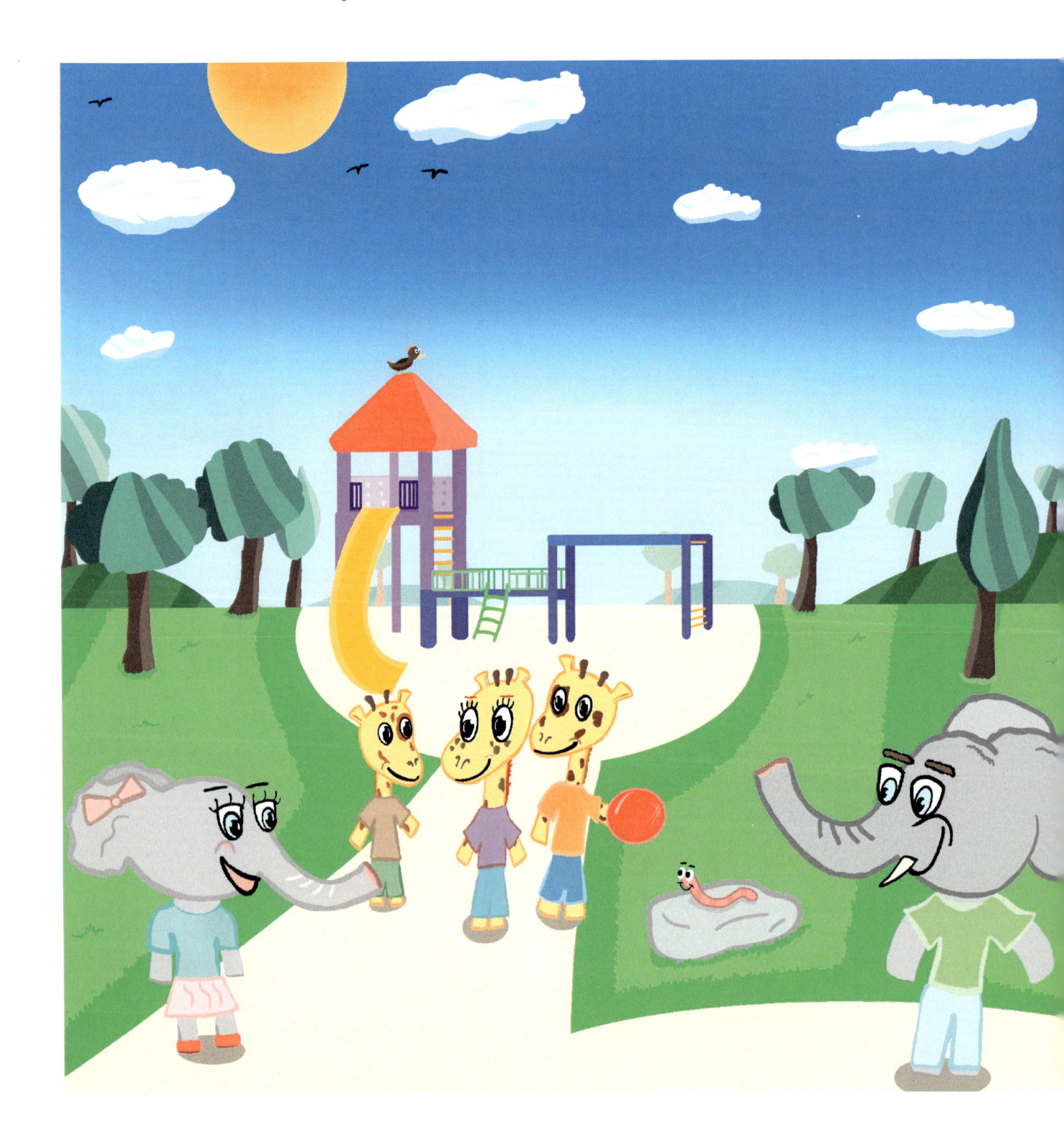

Play and play is what we do!

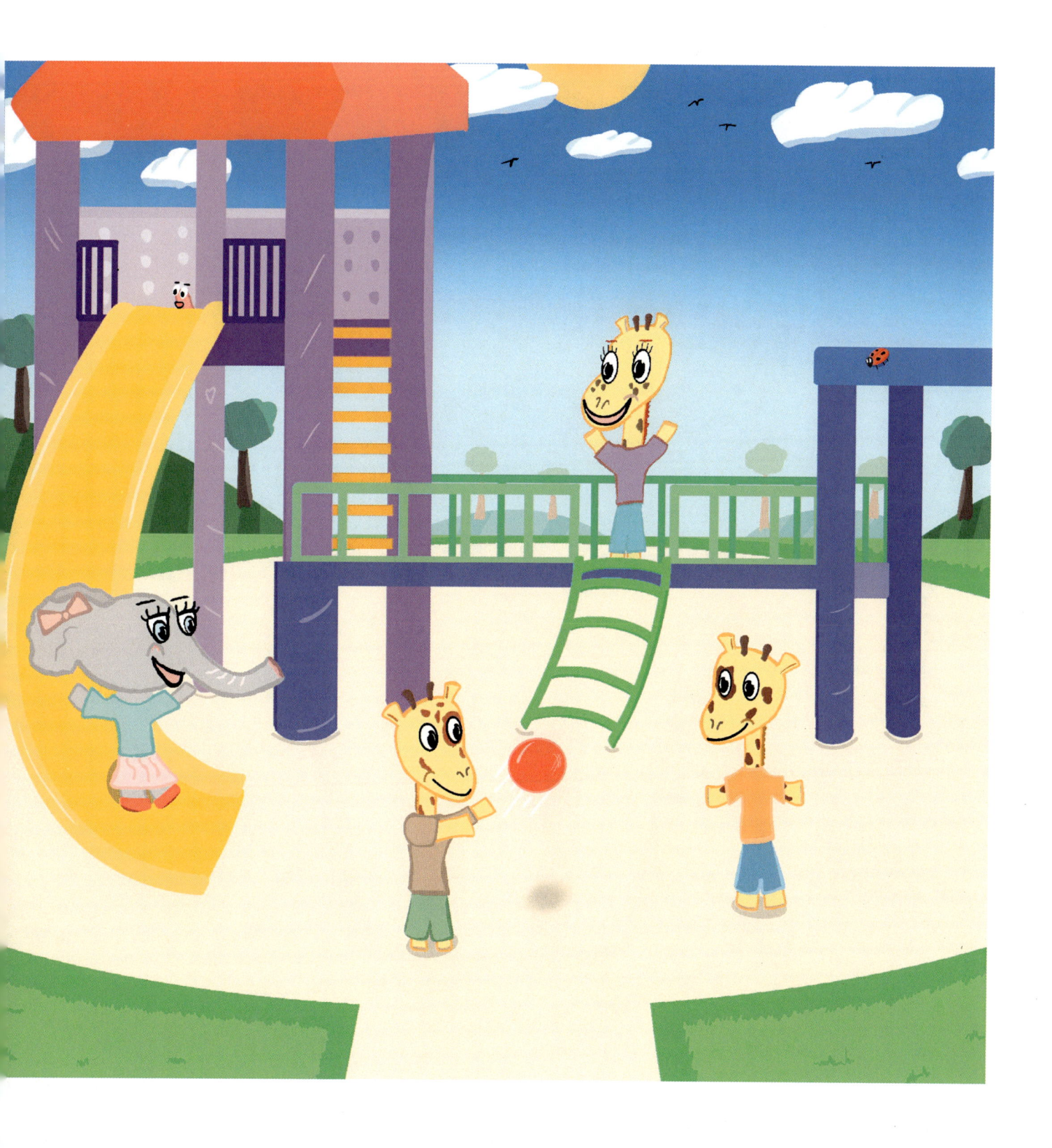

They even just fed me a peanut, too.

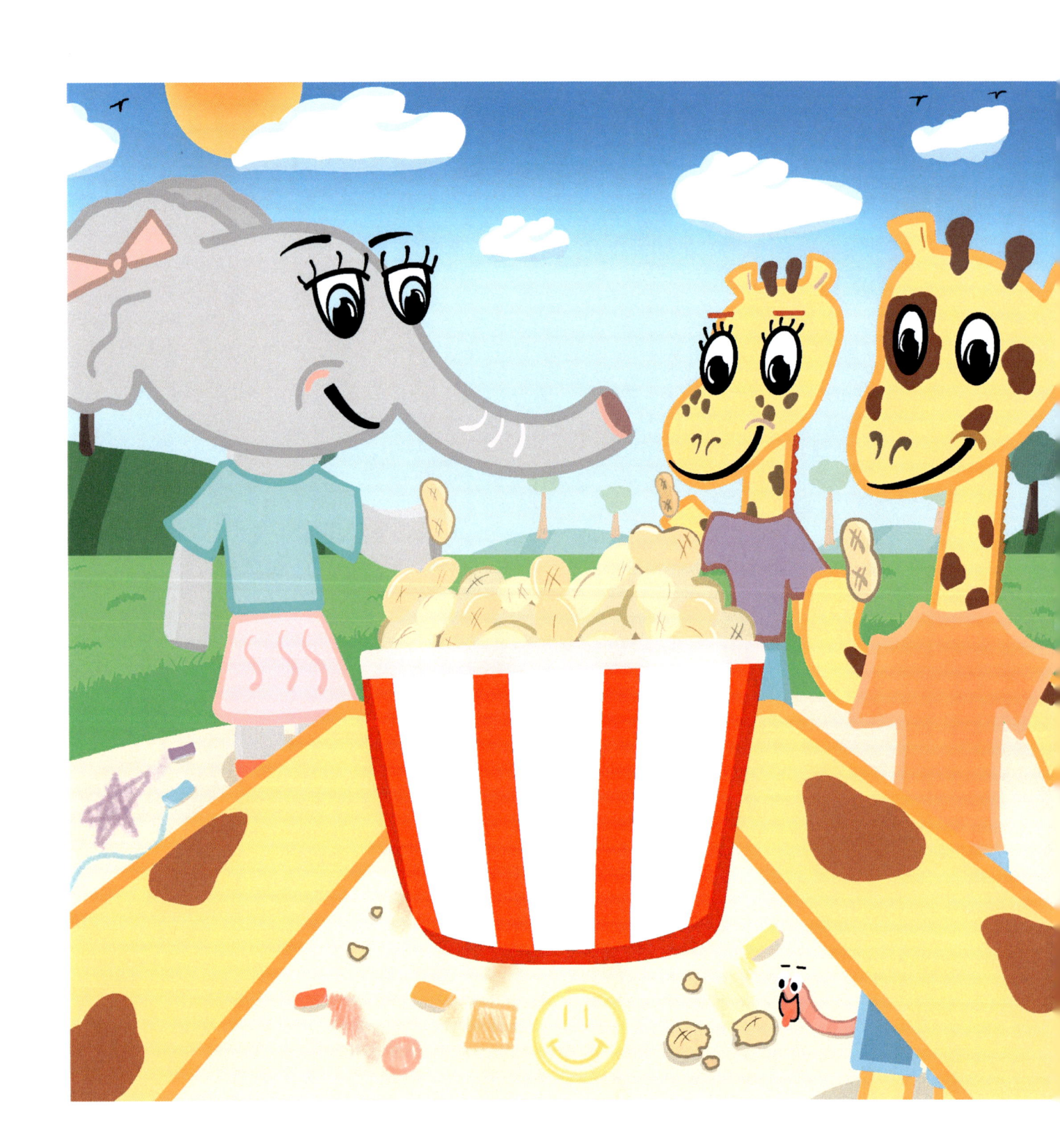

Not feeling well because allergic to peanuts is what I am.

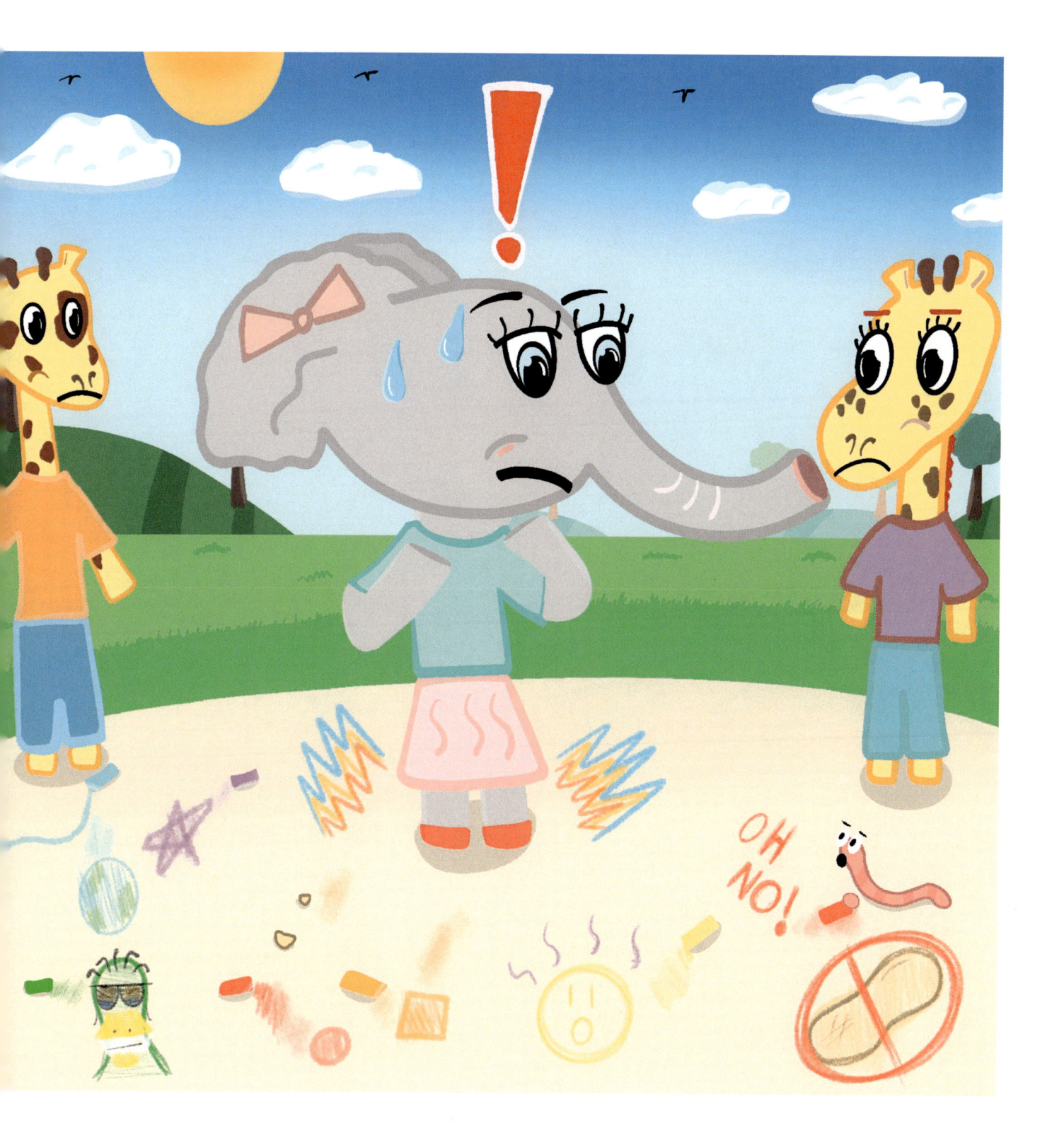

My throat is closing, and I have hives! Call Nurse Pam!

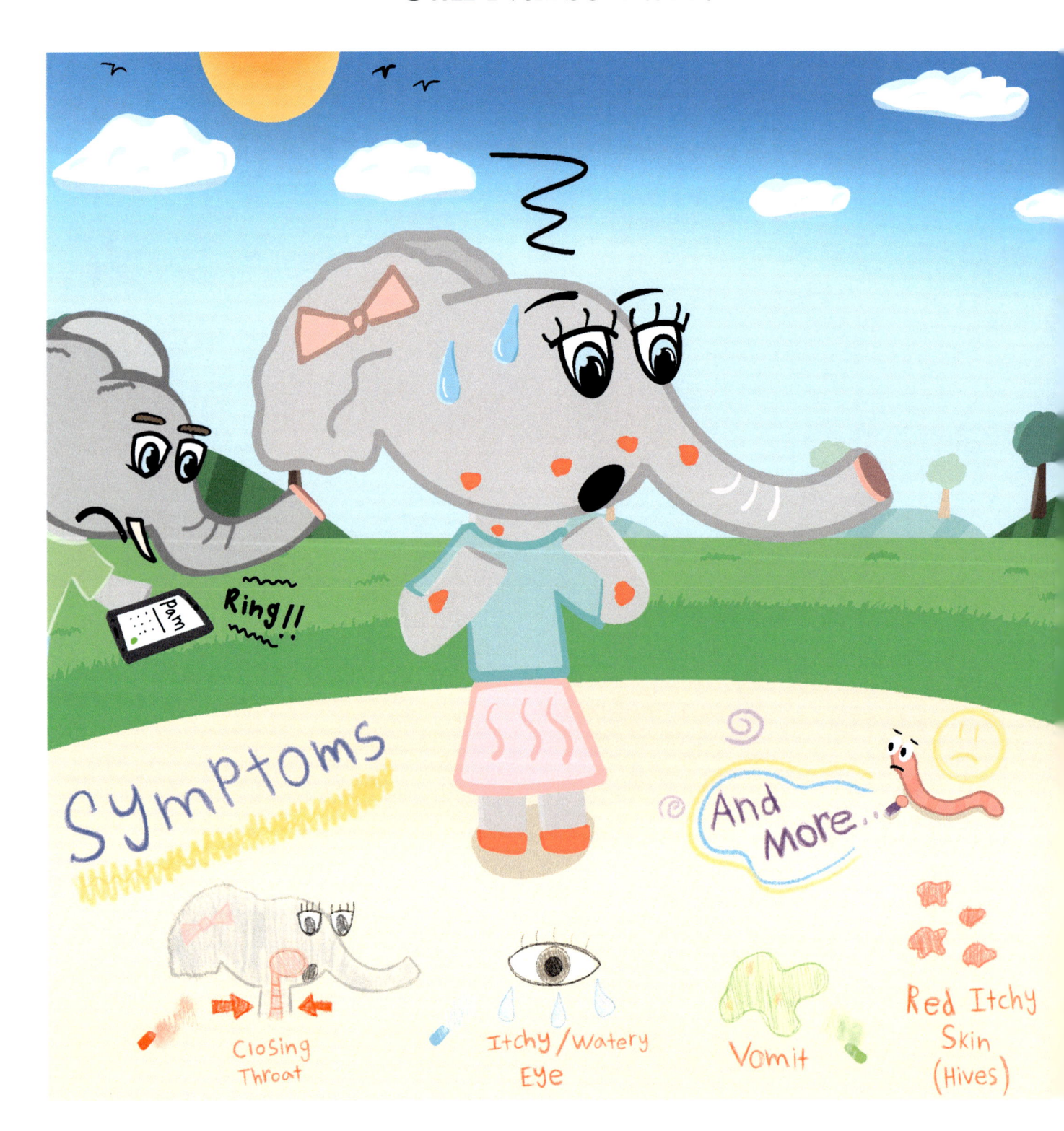

Nurse Pam brings over a special pen.

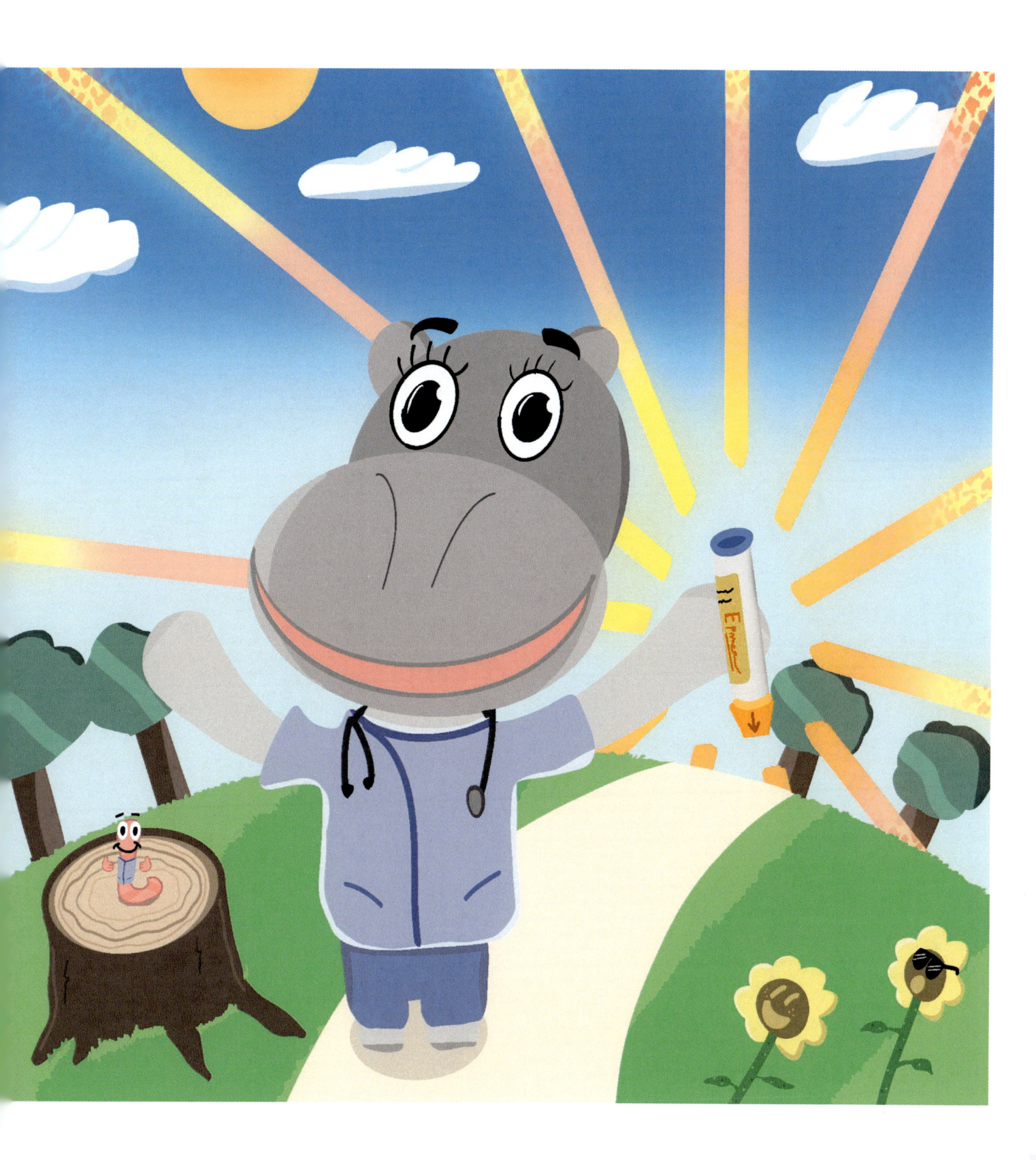

She says it has epi-neph-rine.

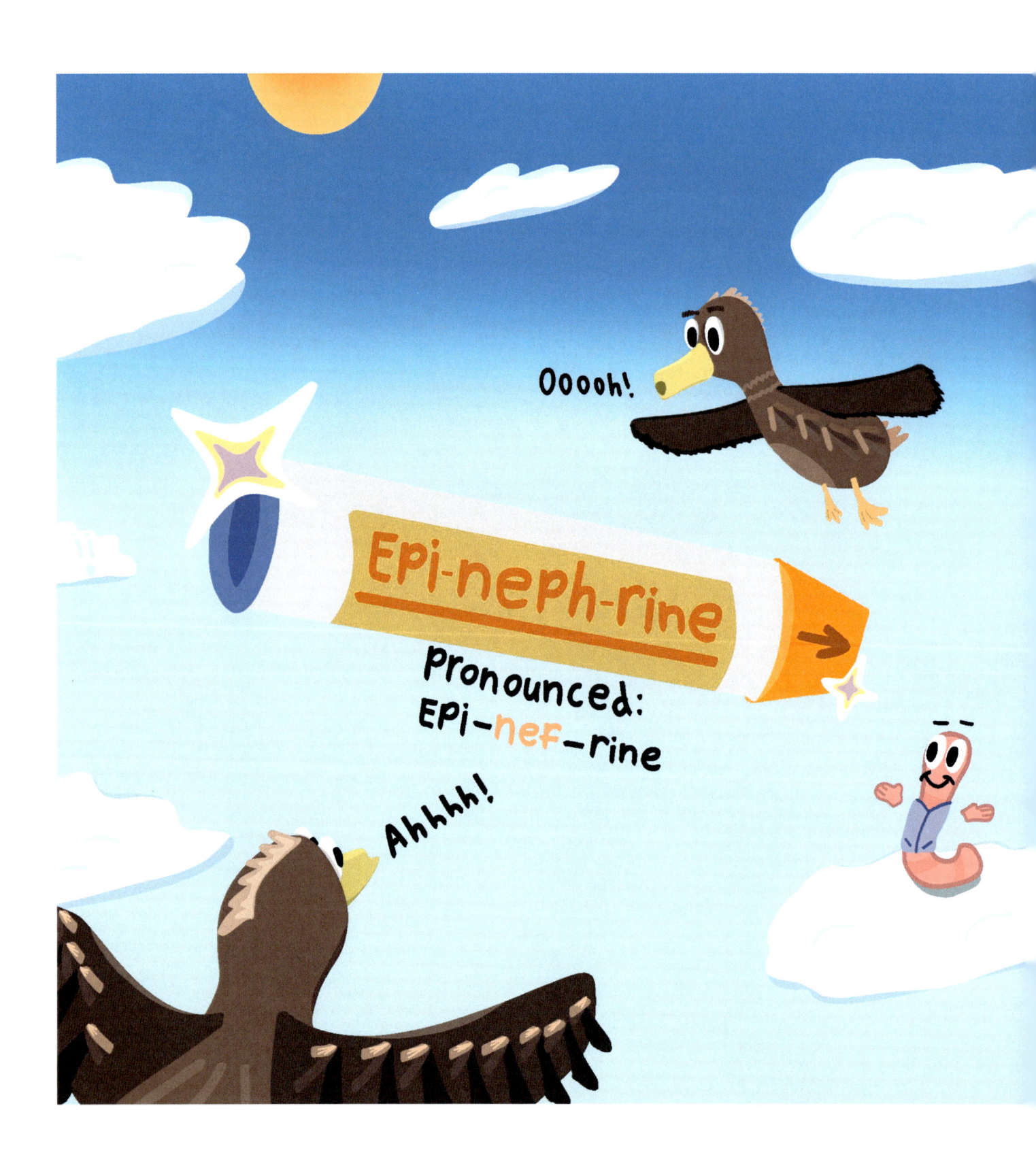

Nurse Pam says:

"I'm going to inject this in your thigh …

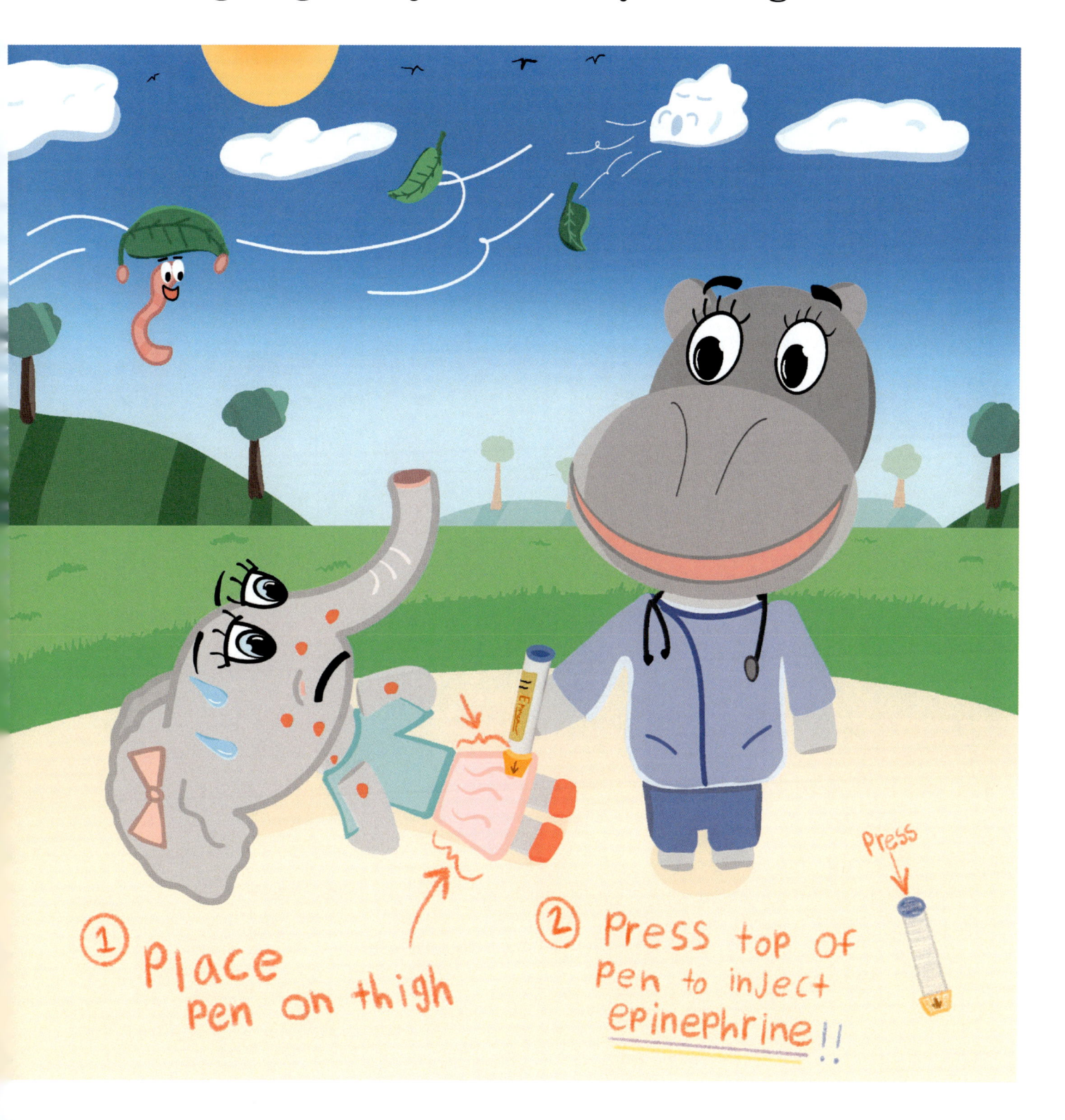

① Place pen on thigh

② Press top of pen to inject epinephrine!!

Press

… then you're closing throat and hives will go
bye-bye."

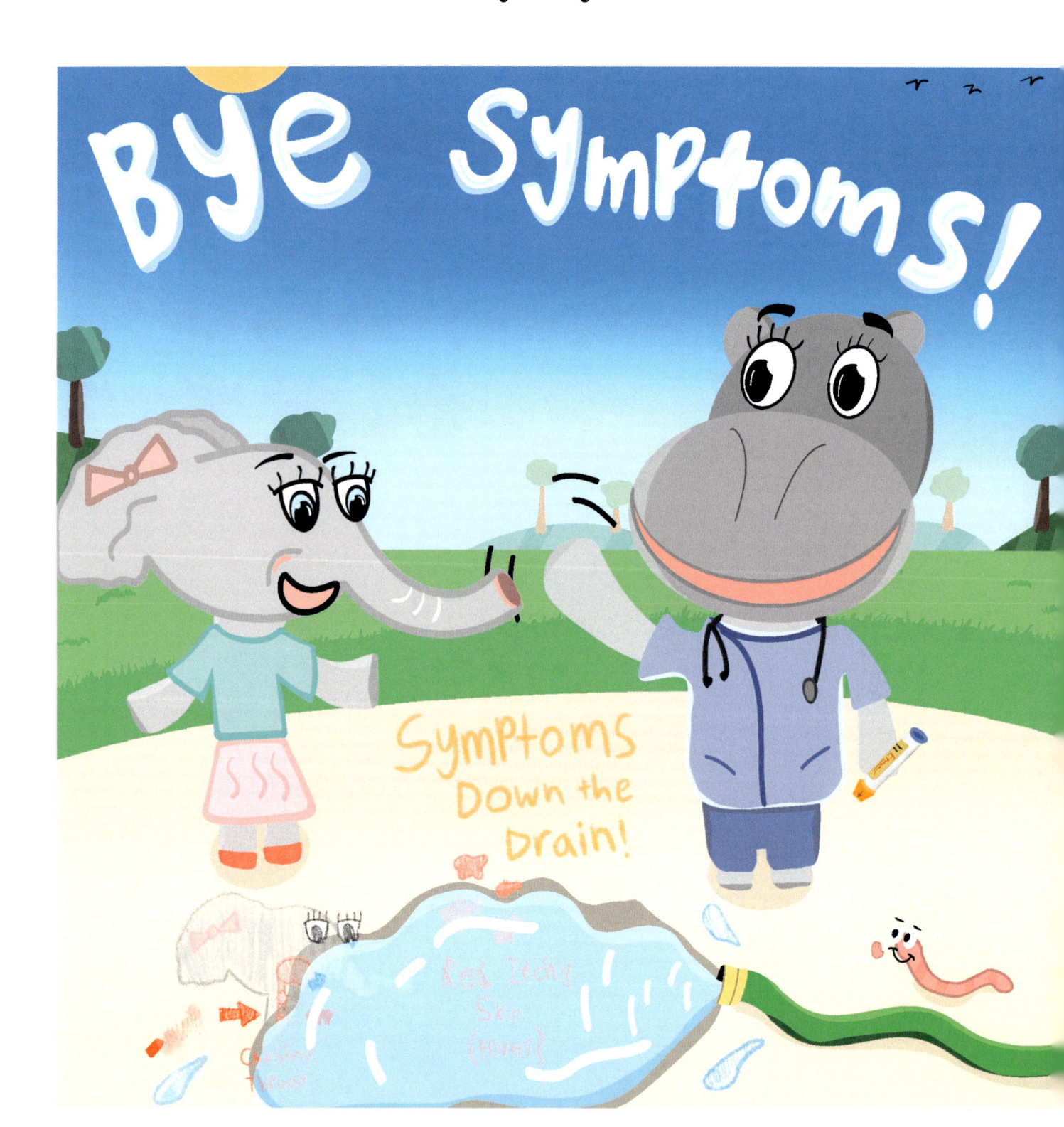

It worked so quickly; that was fast!

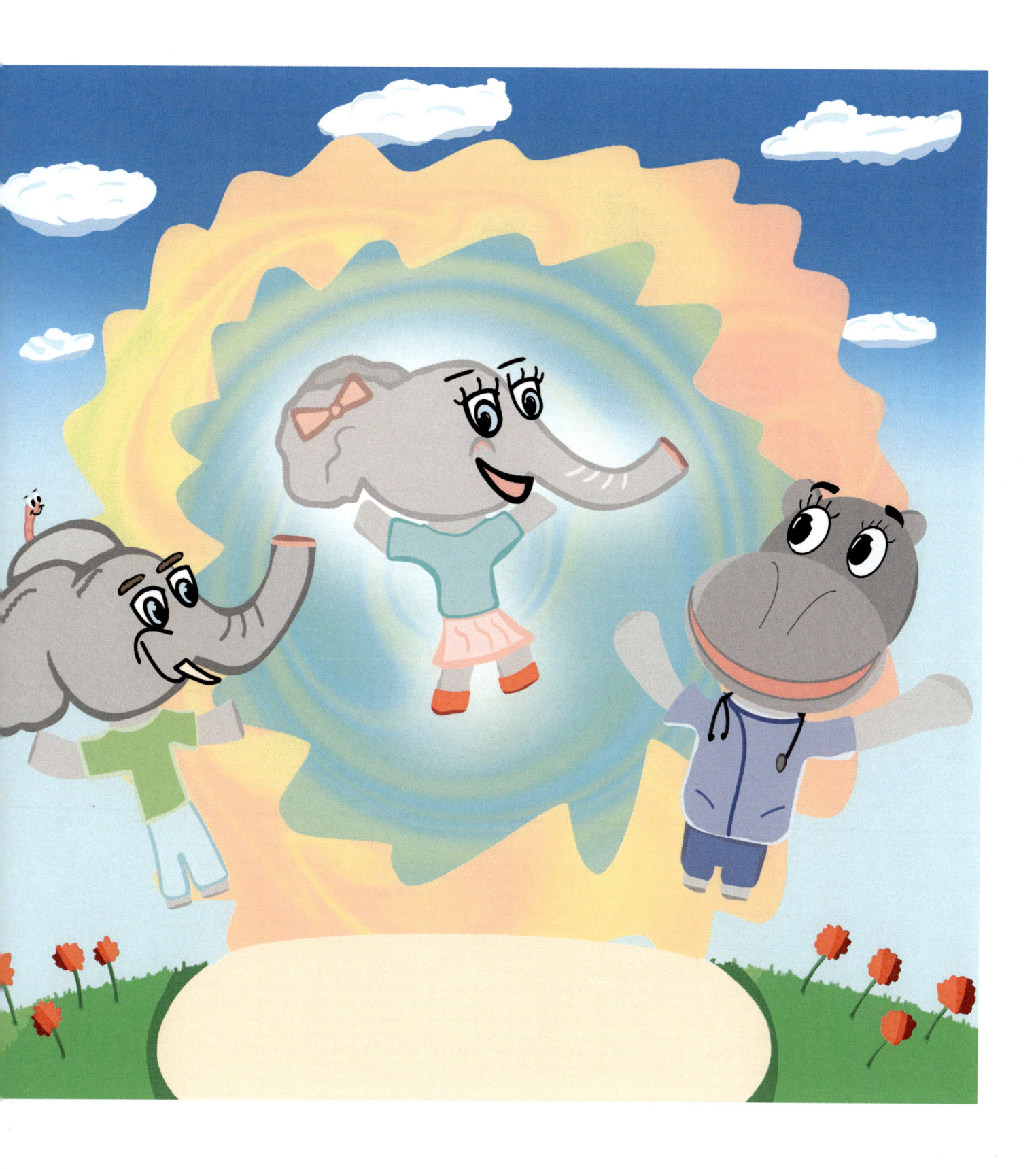

Now I can go back, play with my friends, and have a blast!

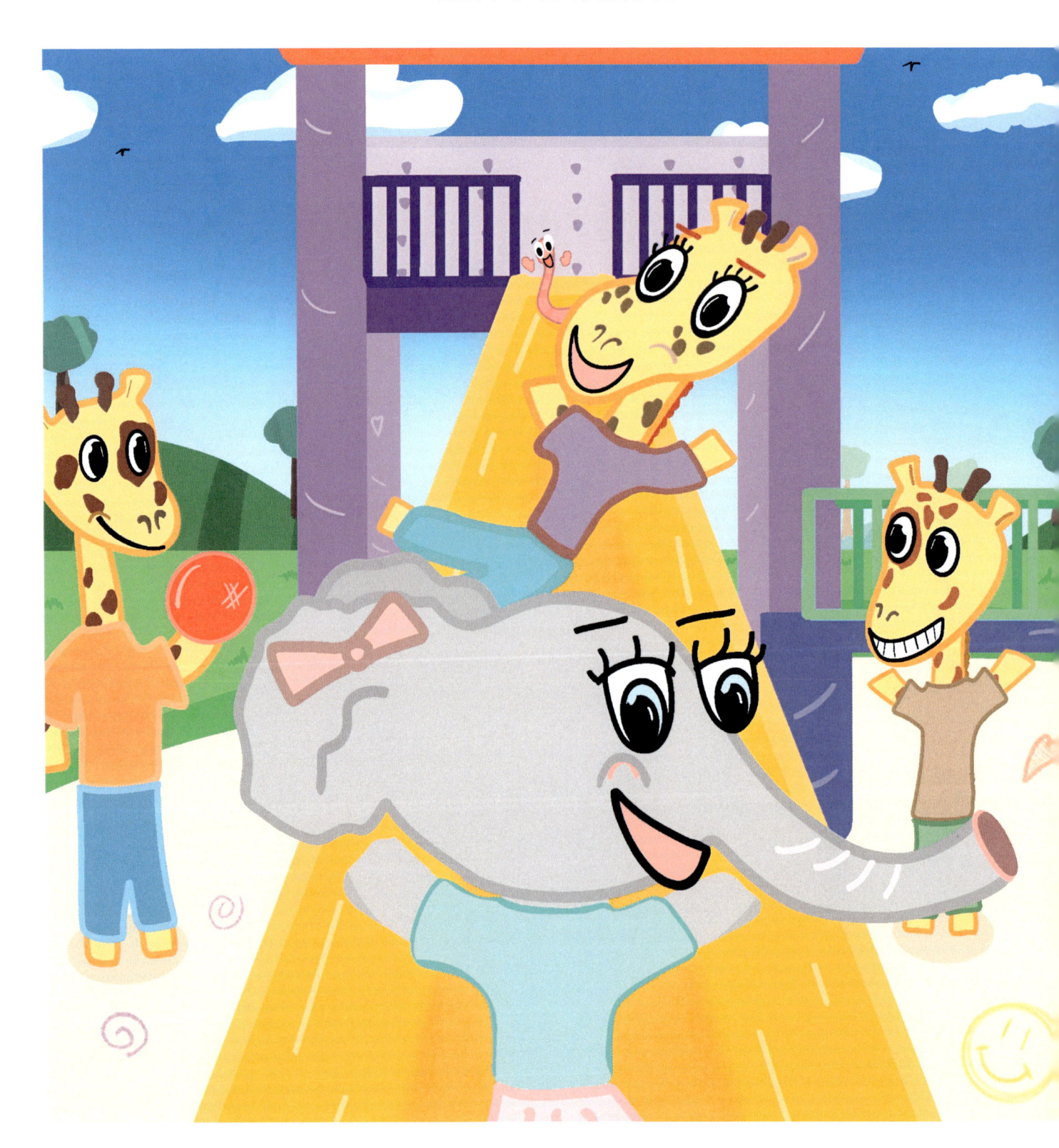

The End!

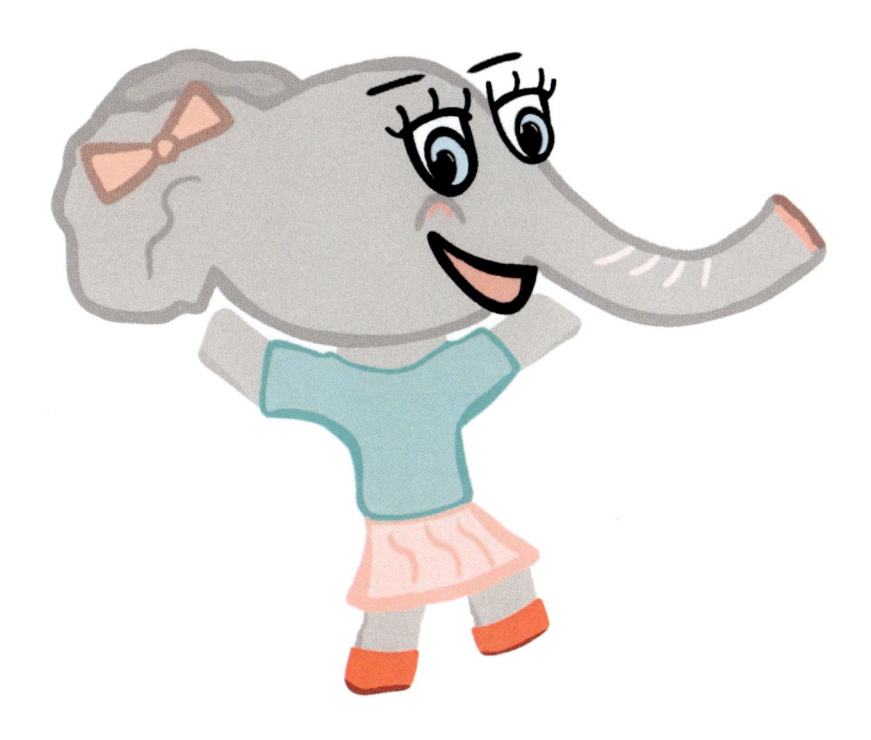

Check out Dr. Willett's other books!

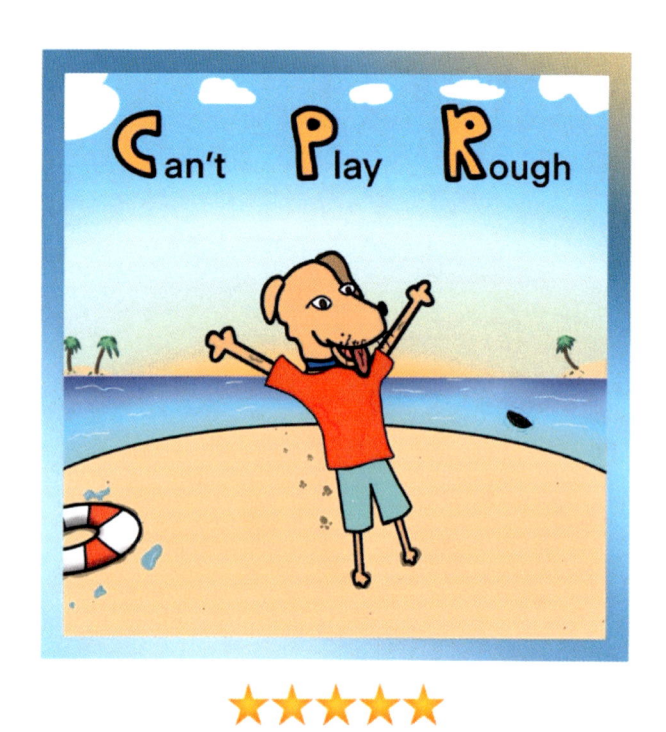

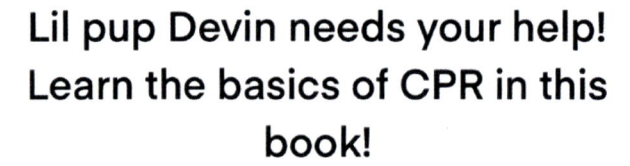

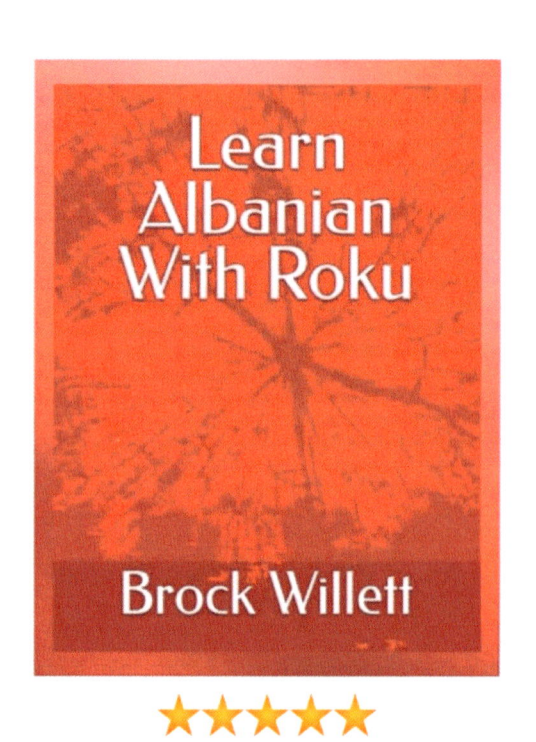

★★★★★   ★★★★★

Lil pup Devin needs your help! Learn the basics of CPR in this book!

Scan For Website!

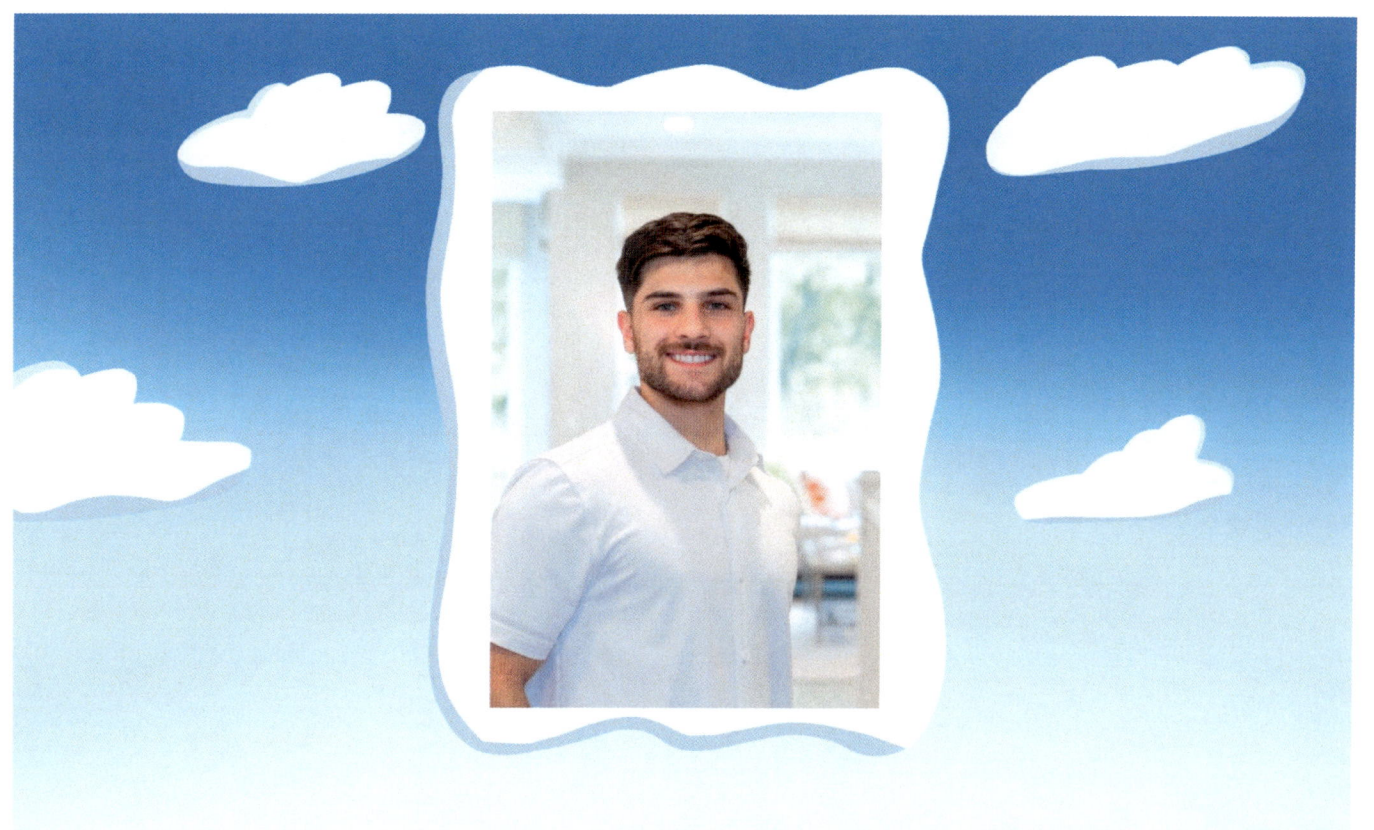

Illustrator Vittorio Nocera is passionate when it comes to making art. Inspired by many of his favorite books during childhood, Vittorio aims to recreate that same magic that once sparked his imagination to help deliver educational messages in fun and colorful ways.

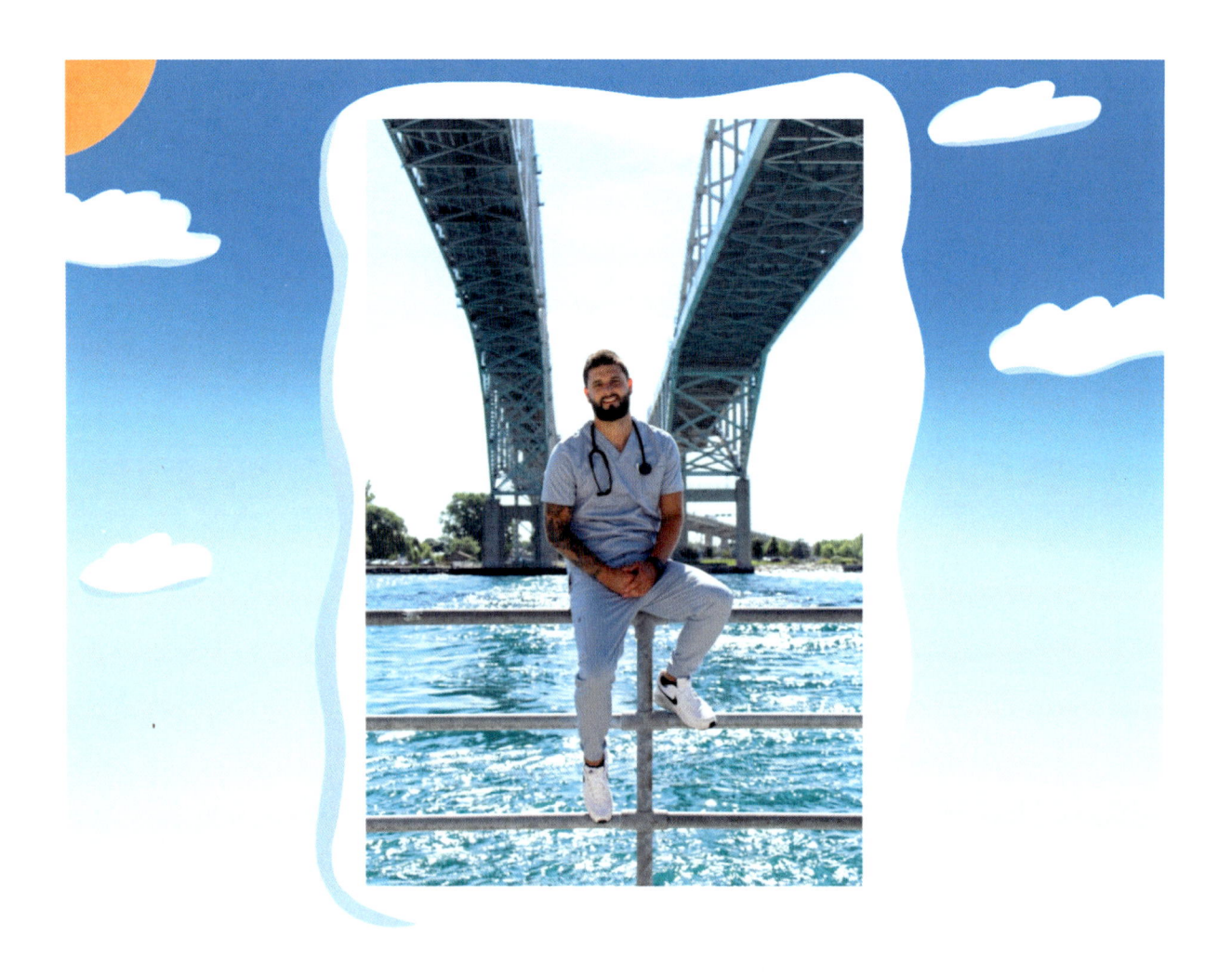

Elephant Playground Incident is the second
children's book written by Brock Willett.
Dr. Willett is passionate about helping children
and parents understand the basics of potentially
life-threatening emergencies.

Made in the USA
Coppell, TX
26 December 2024